50 Ketogenic Diet Recipes
Ketogenic Diet Recipes for Weight Loss

Summary

The Ketogenic Diet has been in existence for at least nine decades. It entails a low carb diet that gives a high fat and moderate protein daily intake. The recipes in this book will help you choose recipes that range from a variety of breakfast, salads, soups, smoothies and many more. In here, you can find what to eat and what to expect to eat as well. Being able to eat a healthy and balanced meal is one of the keys to weight loss, which can aid lessen the risk of diabetes, heart diseases and even some cancers!

This book contains four chapters that can help you in choosing which recipes you would like to make. This book was designed for easy-to-follow instructions, easy navigation as well as easily available ingredients. If you are having difficulty looking for some of the ingredients listed in a recipe, there are alternatives given you can easily substitute what some cannot find in their local grocery.

So what are you waiting for? Make some of these recipes in your home today!

Disclaimer and Terms of Use:

Effort has been made to ensure that the information in this book is accurate and complete, however, the author and the publisher do not warrant the accuracy of the information, text and graphics contained within the book due to the rapidly changing nature of science, research, known and unknown facts and internet. The Author and the publisher do not hold any responsibility for errors, omissions or contrary interpretation of the subject matter herein. This book is presented solely for motivational and informational purposes only.

Table of Contents

Introduction

Top ketogenic recipes that help lose weight and maintain health. Simple and exciting, the book enumerates around 50 recipes that will enhance your eating experience and simultaneously help you lose weight. From breakfast to dinner recipes, this book has it all!

A ketogenic diet is a high protein, high fat and low carb diet that forces the body to use fat instead of carbohydrate. When the body starts using fat instead of carbohydrate, an instant weight loss is seen. The most amazing part of the ketogenic diet is the deliciousness of the recipes, as you will read through during the course of the book.

Primarily, ketogenic diet was used to treat epilepsy in children. With the elevated levels of ketone bodies in the blood, epileptic seizures are controlled and treated.

Similarly, with elevated levels of ketones in the body, the body is forced to burn fat rather than rely on glucose for energy. This state is called ketosis. This diet primarily focuses on losing weight through the use of this technique.

Beverage Recipes

In this chapter, you will find beverages that are easy to make. All you need are the ingredients, a blender and you're good to go. There is an array of beverages to make from non-alcoholic to alcoholic beverages. They will help make you feel full as well as refreshed while still having a low carb intake. Since some of the recipes contain some alcoholic content, please ensure that you are of age or are sure that you are physically fit to drink alcoholic beverages.

Low Carb Mojito

This is perfect for those long and hot days.
This recipe is perfect for an individual drink.

Ingredients:

7-8 Mint leaves with stems attached
2.5 ounces light rum
Juice of 1 lime
1 tablespoon of low carb sugar syrup

Instructions:

1. Blend all the ingredients together.
2. Serve with some ice.

Low Carb Pina Colada

Whether it's summer or you're having a party, this drink will definitely cool you off. This recipe is proportioned for one glass for one person.

Ingredients:

3 ounces of rum
1/2 cup sugar-free pineapple syrup
2 cups crushed ice
2/3 cup coconut milk or cream (make sure it's sugar free)

Instructions:

1. Blend all the ingredients together.
2. Serve.

Blueberry Martini

Here is how to make one serving of this ketogenic delight at home:

Ingredients:

6-7 fresh blueberries
2 ounces plain vodka
2 ounces of blueberry flavored vodka
1 teaspoon of low carb sugar syrup
A few cubes of ice

Instructions:

1. Shake all the ingredients in a shaker.
2. Pour contents without the ice.
3. Serve with blueberries, if desired.

Apple Martini

Here is how to make one serving of this ketogenic delight at home:

Ingredients:

Apple slice
2 ounces plain vodka
2 ounces of apple flavored vodka
1 teaspoon of low carb sugar syrup
A few cubes of ice

Instructions:

1. Shake all the ingredients in a shaker.
2. Pour contents without the ice.
3. Serve with apple slices, if desired.

Low Carb Margarita

Here is how to make one serving of this ketogenic delight at home:

Ingredients:

1.5 ounces of tequila
1/4 teaspoon of orange extract
1/4 cup prepared lemon lime Crystal Light
Crushed ice
2 ounces lime juice

Instructions:

1. Blend all the ingredients together.
2. Serve.

White Chocolate Almond Protein Shake

Here is how to make one glass of this ketogenic delight at home:

Ingredients:

16 ounces unsweetened almond milk

1 tablespoon of Sugar Free White Chocolate syrup

1/2 cup crushed ice (optional: add if you like a thick drink, but the flavor will be less intense.)

4 ounces heavy cream

2 scoops Vanilla Powder

Instructions:

1. Add in all the ingredients in a blender.
2. Blend and serve.

Orange Coconut Protein Shake

Here is how to make one glass of this ketogenic shake at home:

Ingredients:

16 ounces unsweetened almond milk

1 tablespoon of sugar-free Coconut Syrup

1/2 cup crushed ice (optional: add if you like a thick drink, but the flavor will be less intense.)

4 ounces heavy cream

2 scoops Tropical Whey Powder

Instructions:

1. Add in all the ingredients in a blender.
2. Blend and serve.

Chocolate Raspberry Protein Shake

Here is how to make one glass of this ketogenic shake at home:

Ingredients:

16 ounces unsweetened almond milk
1/2 cup crushed ice
4 ounces heavy cream
2 scoops Chocolate powder
1 tablespoon of Sugar Free Raspberry Syrup

Instructions:

1. Add in all the ingredients in a blender.
2. Blend and serve.

Cream and Soda Sparkler

This sparkler will make your taste buds jump with every sip. This recipe should yield two glasses.

Ingredients:

2 ounces heavy cream
Sparkling flavored water, such as La Croix berry flavor (make sure it is unsweetened)
1-2 tablespoons sugar free Raspberry Syrup

Instructions:

1. Add in all the ingredients in a blender.
2. Blend and make sure the mixture is consistent. Serve.

Blueberry Almond Smoothie

Here is how to make this ketogenic delight for one at home.

Ingredients:

16 ounces unsweetened almond milk
4 ounces heavy cream
1/4 cup frozen unsweetened blueberries
1 scoop vanilla powder
1 packet artificial sweetener

Instructions:

1. Add in all the ingredients in a blender.
2. Blend and make sure the mixture is consistent. Serve.

Orange Cooler

Here is how to make this ketogenic delight for one at home.

Ingredients:

16 ounces unsweetened almond milk
4 ounces heavy cream
A few drops of liquid orange extract
1 packet artificial sweetener
1/2 cup crushed ice (optional: add if you like a thick drink, but the flavor will be less intense.)

Instructions:

1. Add in all the ingredients in a blender.
2. Blend and make sure the mixture is consistent. Serve.

Low Carb Strawberry Almond Smoothie

Here is how to make this ketogenic delight for one at home.

Ingredients:

16 ounces unsweetened almond milk
4 ounces heavy cream
1/4 cup frozen unsweetened strawberries
1 scoop vanilla powder
1 packet artificial sweetener

Instructions:

1. Add in all the ingredients in a blender.
2. Blend and make sure the mixture is consistent. Serve.

Low Carb Creamy Chocolate Milk

Here is how to make this ketogenic delight at home. This will serve around 4 people.

Ingredients:

16 ounces unsweetened almond milk
4 ounces heavy cream
1 scoop chocolate powder
1/2 cup crushed ice (optional: add if you like a thick drink, but the flavor will be less intense.)
1 packet artificial sweetener

Instructions:

1. Add in all the ingredients in a blender.
2. Blend and make sure the mixture is consistent. Serve.

Salad Recipes

Salads can be paired with anything and may even be considered as an appetizer. It is great to accompany with main dishes as well as it is also good by itself. With the salad recipes you will find, you can pair it up with any of the quiche recipes in the next chapter of this book.

Egg Salad

Here is how to make this ketogenic delight for around six people, at home:

Ingredients:

12 large hard boiled eggs, sliced
1/2 teaspoon ground mustard
1 teaspoon salt
1/2 cup mayonnaise
2 tablespoons of melted butter
1/3 cup finely minced white onion
1 teaspoon black pepper

Instructions:

1. Add in all the ingredients in a bowl.
2. Toss lightly.
3. Serve.

Tomato and Avocado Salad

Here is how to make this ketogenic salad for four people at home:

Ingredients:

8 ounces ripe tomatoes cut into 1-inch chunks

2 tablespoons mayonnaise

1/4 teaspoon onion powder or 2 ounces finely minced onion

Salt to taste

1 medium ripe Haas Avocado, scooped from shell, and cut into cubes

Instructions:

1. Add all the ingredients in a salad bowl. Toss lightly.
2. Serve.

Spinach and Apple Salad

Here is how to make two to three servings of this ketogenic delight at home:

Ingredients:

3 to 4 cups washed baby spinach leaves
3-4 tablespoons crumbled blue cheese
1/2 small apple, cut into 1/4 inch cubes
1/2 cup thinly sliced red onion

Instructions:

1. Plate the ingredients.
2. Drizzle with your choice of low fat salad dressing. Use around two tablespoons.
3. Toss and serve.

Basic Spinach Salad

Here is how to make two to three servings of this ketogenic delight at home:

Ingredients:

3 to 4 cups washed baby spinach leaves
1/4 cup slivered almonds or chopped macadamia nuts
1/2 cup cooked and crumbled bacon
1/2 cup thinly sliced red onion
3-4 tablespoons crumbled blue cheese

Instructions:

1. Plate the ingredients.
2. Drizzle with your choice of low fat salad dressing (around 2 tablespoons).
3. Toss and serve.

Curried Chicken Salad

Here is how to make two servings of this ketogenic delight at home:

Ingredients:

2 cups diced, cooked chicken breast
1/4 cup sliced almonds
1/4 cup diced jicama
1/2 cup diced celery
2 tablespoons butter
1 raw, organic egg yolk, preferably from pastured chickens (makes for richer, tastier yolk)
2 ounces mayonnaise
1 teaspoon curry powder
1/4 teaspoon stevia glyceride
2 teaspoons lemon juice
1/2 teaspoon salad

Instructions:

1. Toss the first four ingredients in a salad bowl.
2. Cook the rest of the ingredients in a pan for two to three minutes with butter over medium heat. It should form a nice consistent mixture.

3. Transfer it to a bowl and let it cool a little.
4. Toss the sauce with the rest of the ingredients in the salad bowl and serve.

Chicken, Bacon and Tomato Salad

Here is how to make one serving of this ketogenic salad at home:

Ingredients:

1 large uncooked chicken breast, cut into 1 inch chunks
5 slices bacon
Small tomato, seeded and cut into small chunks
2 ounces Muenster cheese, shredded
2 teaspoons Canadian Steak Seasoning
2 tablespoons butter

Instructions:

1. Sprinkle the chicken with the Canadian Steak seasoning.
2. Cook the chicken in a skillet with the butter on medium heat, ten minutes one each side. Plate.
3. In the same skillet, cook the bacon strips. Tap the bacon strips to get rid of the extra grease. Chop the chicken and bacon into bite size.
4. Combine the tomatoes, chicken and bacon. Squeeze in a bit of lemon or as

desired. Sprinkle some cheese on top before serving.

Pineapple Fruit Salad

Here is how to make around one glass of this ketogenic delight at home:

Ingredients:

1 cup of raw raspberries (8.4 net carbs)
1/2 cup of raw blueberries (8.6 net carbs)
1/2 cup raw pineapple (8.7 net carbs)

Instructions:

1. Chop the ingredients.
2. Add in a salad bowl; squeeze half a lemon, if wanted. Toss lightly.
3. Serve.

Honeydew Melon Salad

Here is how to make one serving of this ketogenic delight at home:

Ingredients:

1/2 cup raw honeydew melon (7.8 net carbs)
1 raw lime (7.1 net carbs)
1 medium tangerine (9.4 net carbs)

Instructions:

1. Chop the ingredients.
2. Add in a salad bowl; squeeze half a lemon, if wanted. Toss lightly.
3. Serve.

Valencia Orange Salad

Here is how to make one serving of this ketogenic delight at home:

Ingredients:

1 raw plum (8.6 net carbs)
1/2 medium apple (9.0 net carbs)
1/2 Valencia orange (5.2 net carbs)

Instructions:

1. Chop the ingredients.
2. Add in a salad bowl and toss lightly.
3. Serve.

Fruit Salad with Less Than Five Net Carbs

Here is how to make two servings of this ketogenic delight at home:

Ingredients:

1/2 cup of raw strawberries (3.3 net carbs)
5 whole sweet cherries (5.1 net carbs)
1/2 of a kiwi fruit (4.3 net carbs)
1 medium apricot (3.2 net carbs)
1/2 cup of raw raspberries (4.2 net carbs)
1/2 of a medium peach (4.3 net carbs)

Instructions:

1. Chop and serve all the ingredients on a plate.
2. Toss and serve.

Main Course Recipes

The main courses in this chapter consist mostly of quiche. Quiche is healthy and can be served for breakfast, lunch, brunch or dinner. Beyond this, it contains essential vitamins and minerals needed by the body.

Basic Quiche Recipe

Here is how to make this ketogenic delight at home and serve around four people.

Ingredients:

5-6 cups Colby jack cheese, divided in half
2 cups heavy cream
1 tsp salt
1 tsp ground black pepper
2 tsp dried thyme
2 tablespoons butter
1 large white onion, finely chopped
12 large eggs, preferably organic or free range eggs

Instructions:

1. Preheat oven to 350 F (175 C).
2. Whisk all the ingredients together.
3. Grease quiche pans.
4. Bake for 20 minutes until the top browns.

One Skillet Bacon and Eggs

Here is how to make this ketogenic delight at home for one person.

Ingredients:

1 tablespoon butter
½ cup finely chopped celery
½ large white onion, chopped into small pieces
4 large organic eggs
½ cup shredded Colby jack cheese
8 slices meaty bacon
1 carrot, peeled into thin strips
½ cup chopped broccoli or cauliflower

Instructions:

1. Heat butter in a skillet.
2. Add in the veggies and the eggs with the bacon.
3. Sprinkle cheese when the eggs are done.
4. Serve.

Peppery Yellow Squash

Here is how to make this ketogenic delight for four to six people:

Ingredients:

- 1/2 of a large white onion, sliced and chopped
- 3-4 tablespoons butter or olive oil
- 2 teaspoons black pepper
- salt to taste
- 1/2 cup of shredded Colby jack cheese
- 5 cups yellow squash, quartered and sliced

Instructions:

1. Start by heating some butter in a skillet over medium heat. Then add the onions, followed by the rest of the ingredients. (Don't add the Colby jack yet. It will be added at the end.)
2. Cover and cook until the squash softens. This should take around ten minutes.
3. Sprinkle some Colby jack on top and serve.

Yellow Squash With Basil

Here is how to make this ketogenic delight for four to six people:

Ingredients:

- 1 tablespoon julienned fresh basil leaves
- 1 clove garlic, minced
- 3 tablespoons butter or olive oil
- 4 cups yellow squash, quartered and sliced
- salt to taste
- 1 tablespoon lemon juice (to be added at the end)

Instructions:

1. Start by heating some butter in a skillet over medium heat. Then add the onions, followed by the rest of the ingredients.
2. Cover and cook until the squash softens, this should take around 10 minutes.
3. Squeeze the lemon on top and serve.

Cauliflower Casserole

Here is how to make this ketogenic delight for four to six people:

Ingredients:

- 2 lb. raw cauliflower, trimmed of leaves and lower stalk
- 4 ounces chopped white onion
- 4 fl oz. heavy cream
- 4 oz. cream cheese
- 2 cups shredded Colby jack or cheddar
- 1 tablespoon butter
- 2 ounces chicken broth

Instructions:

1. Preheat the oven at 350 F (175 C).
2. Add all the ingredients a skillet, except for cheese.
3. Transfer in a casserole with cheese on top to a preheated oven for 20 minutes.
4. Serve.

Cauliflower and Bacon Quiche

Here is how to make this ketogenic delight at home:

Ingredients:

2 lb raw cauliflower, trimmed of leaves and lower stalk
4 ounces minced white onion
4 ounces cooked and crumbled bacon
2 cups shredded colby jack or cheddar
6 eggs
1/2 cup heavy cream
Salt and pepper to taste
2 ounces minced green pepper
1 tablespoon butter

Instructions:

1. Preheat oven to 350 degrees (175 C).
2. Whisk all the ingredients together until all the ingredients distribute evenly.
3. Grease quiche pans
4. Bake for 20 minutes
5.

Pickling Spice

Here is how to make this ketogenic delight for three to four people at home:

Ingredients:

2 tablespoons butter
1 yellow onion, chopped
3 cloves garlic, minced
2 teaspoon chili powder
1 teaspoon ground coriander
1/2 cup sour cream
2 to 3 cups grated Monterey Jack cheese or cheddar cheese
1 pound ground beef
4 oz. can of green chilies
2 teaspoons ground cumin
Six baked tart crust

Instructions:

1. Mix in all the ingredients in a bowl.
2. Cook in a skillet for five minutes.
3. Spoon into baked tart crusts.
4. Bake for ten minutes in a preheated oven at 350 F (175 C).
5. Serve.

Cheese and Onion Quiche with Sausage

Here is how to make this ketogenic quiche for three to four people at home:

Ingredients:

5-6 cups shredded Muenster and/or Colby jack cheese, divided in half

2 tablespoons butter plus more for greasing pans

2 sausages, diced

2 cups heavy cream

12 large eggs, preferably organic or free range eggs

1 tsp salt

1 tsp ground black pepper

2 tsp dried thyme

1 large white onion, finely chopped

Instructions:

1. Preheat oven to 350 F (175 C).
2. Whisk all the ingredients together until all the ingredients distribute evenly.
3. Grease quiche pans.
4. Bake for 20 minutes.

Veggie Quiche

Here is how to make this ketogenic quiche for three to four people at home:

Ingredients:

- 12 large eggs, preferably organic or free range eggs
- 1 tsp salt
- 1 tsp ground black pepper
- 2 tsp dried thyme
- 1 large white onion, finely chopped
- 5-6 cups shredded Muenster and/or Colby jack cheese, divided in half
- 2 tablespoons butter plus more for greasing pans
- 2 cups heavy cream
- Diced vegetable of your choice

Instructions:

1. Preheat oven to 350 F (175 C).
2. Whisk all the ingredients together until all the ingredients distribute evenly.
3. Grease quiche pans.
4. Bake for 20 minutes.

Bacon Quiche

Here is how to make this ketogenic quiche for three to four people at home:

Ingredients:

5-6 cups shredded Muenster and/or Colby jack cheese, divided in half

2 tablespoons butter plus more for greasing pans

5 slices of bacon, diced

2 cups heavy cream

2 tsp dried thyme

1 large white onion, finely chopped

12 large eggs, preferably organic or free range eggs

1 tsp salt

1 tsp ground black pepper

Instructions:

1. Preheat oven to 350 F (175 C).
2. Whisk all the ingredients together until all the ingredients distribute evenly.
3. Grease quiche pans.
4. Bake for 20 minutes.

Kitchen Sink Quiche

Here is how to make this ketogenic quiche for three to four people at home:

Ingredients:

5-6 cups shredded Muenster and/or Colby jack cheese, divided in half
2 tablespoons butter plus more for greasing pans
5 slices of bacon, diced
2 cups heavy cream
2 tsp dried thyme
1 large white onion, finely chopped
12 large eggs, preferably organic or free range eggs
1 tsp salt
A handful of chopped veggies of your choice
2 sausages, diced
1 tsp ground black pepper

Instructions:

1. Preheat oven to 350 F (175 C).
2. Whisk all the ingredients together until all the ingredients distribute evenly.
3. Grease quiche pans.
4. Bake for 20 minutes.

Baked Salmon

Here is how to make around two servings of this ketogenic delight at home:

Ingredients:

2 cloves garlic, minced
6 tablespoons light olive oil
1 teaspoon ground black pepper
1 tablespoon lemon juice
1 tablespoon fresh parsley, chopped
2 (6 ounce) salmon fillets
1 teaspoon dried basil
1 teaspoon salt

Instructions:

1. Preheat oven to 350 F (175 C).
2. Marinate the salmon with all the mentioned ingredients.
3. Bake for 10 minutes.

Herb Baked Salmon

Here is how to make around two servings of this ketogenic delight at home:

Ingredients:

2 pounds salmon fillets

4 ounces sesame oil

1/2 cup tamari soy sauce

1 teaspoon minced garlic

1/2 teaspoon ground ginger

1/2 teaspoon basil

1/4 teaspoon tarragon

4 ounces butter

1/2 cup chopped fresh mushrooms

1/2 cup chopped green onions

1 teaspoon oregano leaves

1/4 teaspoon thyme

1/2 teaspoon rosemary

Instructions:

1. Preheat oven to 350 F (175 C).
2. Marinate the salmon with all the mentioned ingredients.
3. Bake for 10 minutes in the oven.

Chicken in Herb Sauce

Here is how to make this ketogenic delight for two to three servings at home:

Ingredients:

5 tablespoons butter, divided
2 small white onions, thinly sliced
3 large garlic cloves
½ cup chicken broth
½ cup dry white wine
1 ½ tsp Herbs De Provence
1 tsp Chicken Seasoning
Salt to taste
4 raw chicken breasts
8 oz. cream cheese
½ cup heavy cream
1 tsp dried tarragon

Instructions:

1. In a skillet add the butter and the rest of the ingredients; add the cream at the end after the chicken is done. The chicken should be done in a total of twenty minutes, 10 minutes on each side.
2. Serve.

Beef Stew Seasoning

Here is how to make two servings of this ketogenic delight at home:

Ingredients:

2-3 tablespoons butter
4 ounces of white onion, chopped fine
3 garlic cloves, minced
4 boneless, skinless, chicken breast halves
2- 6oz cans diced tomatoes and green chilies
1 teaspoon dried cumin
½ teaspoon garlic powder to taste
1 teaspoon sea salt
4 oz. full fat cream cheese, cut into slices or cubes
¼ cup whipping cream
¼ cup chicken broth
½ teaspoon cayenne pepper (to taste)
Grated cheddar cheese for garnish
Sour cream for garnish
Salsa for garnish

Instructions:

1. In a skillet add the butter and the rest of the ingredients; add the cream at the end after the chicken is done. The chicken should be done in a total of

twenty minutes, 10 minutes on each side.

2. Serve with salsa on top.

Italian Meatballs

Here is how to make two servings of this ketogenic delight at home:

Ingredients:

4 ounces white onion, minced
1 tablespoon olive oil
1 cup cold whole milk ricotta cheese
1 cold large egg
1½ teaspoons sea salt
½ tsp freshly ground black pepper
1 cup shredded parmesan/ Asia-go/Romano mix
1 pound ground beef (92 % lean)
1½ teaspoons granulated garlic
2 teaspoons Italian seasoning

Instructions:

1. Preheat oven to 350 F (175 C).
2. In a bowl mix in all the ingredients.
3. Spoon in the mixture on the baking sheet.
4. Bake for 20 minutes.

Snacks, Pastries and Desserts

Nobody wants to miss out on dessert while on a diet. In this chapter, you will find different types of desserts that range from something you just chop up or something you bake. So let's get started on making our desserts.

Peppery Cheese Biscuits

Here is how to make around 6-8 cookies with this ketogenic recipe:

Ingredients:

2 ½ cups almond flour, divided
6 ounces shredded Colby jack cheese
5 tbsp. butter
2 large eggs
3 tsp freshly cracked black pepper (or 2 tsp ground black pepper)
1 tsp baking soda
¾ tsp xanthium gum
1 tsp sea salt
8 oz. cream cheese

Instructions:

1. Preheat oven to 350 F (175 C).
2. In a bowl mix in all the ingredients.
3. Spoon in the mixture on the baking sheet.
4. Bake for 15 minutes.

Cheddar Garlic Biscuits

Here is how to make around 6-8 cookies with this ketogenic recipe:

Ingredients:

2 ½ cups almond flour, divided
6 ounces shredded Colby jack cheese
5 tbsp. butter
2 tsp granulated garlic
1 tsp baking soda
¾ tsp xanthium gum
1 tsp sea salt
8 oz. cream cheese
2 large eggs

Instructions:

1. Preheat oven to 350 F (175 C).
2. In a bowl mix in all the ingredients.
3. Spoon in the mixture on the baking sheet.
4. Bake for 15 minutes.

Peanut Butter Cookies

Here is how to make around 6 cookies with this ketogenic recipe at home:

Ingredients:

4 ounces cream cheese, softened

2 tablespoons butter, room temperature

1 cup unsweetened natural peanut butter, room temperature*

2/3 cup powdered erythritol

1/2 cup Brown Just like Sugar

2 teaspoons pure vanilla extract

1 teaspoon baking soda

1 teaspoon stevia glyceride

5 drops liquid Splenda

2 large eggs

2 cups almond flour

1/8 teaspoon xanthium gum

1/4 teaspoon salt

Instructions:

1. Preheat oven to 350 F (175 C).
2. In a bowl mix in all the ingredients.
3. Spoon in the mixture on the baking sheet.
4. Bake for 15 minutes until the top crisps.

Crab Meat Bites

Here is how to make this ketogenic delight for three to four people at home:

Ingredients:

1 can crab meat, drained and picked over for shells bits

8 ounces cream cheese, softened to room temperature

1/4 cup heavy cream

2 tablespoons finely chopped red bell pepper

1/2 teaspoon salt

1/2 teaspoon dry mustard

1 tablespoon lemon juice

2 tablespoons finely chopped onion

2 tablespoons finely chopped celery

Six baked tart crusts

Instructions:

1. Mix in all the ingredients in a bowl.
2. Spoon into baked tart crusts.
3. Bake for ten minutes in a preheated oven at 350 F (175 C).
4. Serve.

Rich Chocolate Chip Muffins

Here is how to make around ten to twelve muffins with this ketogenic recipe at home:

Ingredients:

- 2 cups Almond Flour
- 1 cup heavy cream
- 1 tsp vanilla extract
- 1 tsp. baking soda
- ¼ tsp. salt
- ½ cup of Semi-Sweet Chocolate Chips
- 2 large eggs
- 1/8 cup melted butter
- 1/4 cup erythritol or xylitol

Instructions:

1. Preheat oven to 350 F (175 C).
2. Start by adding all the dry ingredients and then add the wet ingredients. Use a whisk to avoid lumps.
3. Bake for 15 minutes in a muffin tray. Use a toothpick and check to see if the toothpick turns out dry, which means your muffins are done.

Low Carb Blueberry Lemon Muffins

Here is how to make this ketogenic delight at home. This will serve around 4 people.

Ingredients:

2 cups Almond Flour
1 cup heavy cream
½ tsp. baking soda
½ tsp lemon extract or flavoring
½ tsp dried lemon zest
¼ tsp. salt
4 ounces fresh blueberries
2 eggs
1/8 cup melted butter
5 packets artificial sweetener such as splenda or stevia

Instructions:

4. Preheat oven to 350 F (175 C).
5. Start by adding all the dry ingredients and then add the wet ingredients. Use a whisk to avoid lumps.
6. Bake for 15 minutes in a muffin tray. Use a toothpick and check to see if the toothpick turns out dry, which means your muffins are done.

Berries on a Plate with Grapes

Here is how to make two servings of this ketogenic delight at home:

Ingredients:

1 cup of raw strawberries (6.6 net carbs)
1/2 cup of raw boysenberries (8.0 net carbs)
1/2 cup of blackberries (5.9 net carbs)
1/2 cup raw grapes (7.1 net carbs)

Instructions:

1. Chop the ingredients.
2. Add in a salad bowl and toss lightly.
3. Serve.

Caramel Chocolate Chip Mini Muffins

Here is how to make these ketogenic muffins to serve four to six people at home:

Ingredients:

   2 cups Almond Flour
   1/8 cup erythritol
   2 T butter, melted, and slightly cooled
   1 tsp stevia glycerite
   ½ cup of Caramel Dip
   ¾ cup Semi-Sweet Chocolate Chips
   1/2 tsp baking soda
   1/2 tsp salt
   1/2 tsp xanthan gum
   2 large eggs, lightly beaten
   1 cup sour cream

Instructions:

7. Preheat oven to 350 (175 C).
8. Start by adding all the dry ingredients and then add the wet ingredients. Use a whisk to avoid lumps.
9. Bake for 15 minutes in a muffin tray. Use a toothpick and check to see if the toothpick turns out dry, which means your muffins are done.

Veggie Bites

Here is how to make this ketogenic snack for three to four people at home:

Ingredients:

8 ounces cream cheese, softened to room temperature
1/2 cup heavy cream
1/4 cup finely chopped red bell pepper
1/4 cup finely chopped celery
1/4 cup finely grated carrot
1/4 cup finely chopped broccoli
1 teaspoon salt
1/2 teaspoon seasoned salt
1/2 cup sour cream
1/4 cup finely chopped onion
Six baked tart crust

Instructions:

1. Mix in all the ingredients in a bowl.
2. Spoon into baked tart crusts.
3. Bake for ten minutes in a preheated oven at 350 F (175 C).
4. Serve.

Conclusion

Like you must have read, this book is especially designed for individuals who want to maintain a healthy weight. The recipes are simple and classic. They do not require a lot of work. In a simple few steps, you can easily create your own recipes once you learn the basic of ketogenic diet.

Using these recipes, you will realize how amazingly easy it is to undergo such a diet, because it literally gives you everything you crave, from cheese to meat and fish. Ketogenic recipes can easily become a favorite of kids.

Easy ingredients and easy recipes and you will be able to lose more weight by activating the ketosis in your body. The moment your body starts utilizing fat instead of carbohydrates in the body, your body starts reducing as the adipose tissues start burning, thus, leaving your body lean.

For decades, ketogenic diets have been prescribed to kids with epilepsy. By activating ketosis in such kids, the symptoms of epilepsy were evidently reduced with this ketogenic diet. Now, using the same concept, you can also lose weight.

The recipes are nutritious and healthy. I'm sure your mouth must already be watering. So, what are you waiting for?

Printed in Great Britain
by Amazon.co.uk, Ltd.,
Marston Gate.